FIGHTING EBOLA: A GROUND–LEVEL VIEW

HEARING

BEFORE THE

SUBCOMMITTEE ON AFRICA, GLOBAL HEALTH, GLOBAL HUMAN RIGHTS, AND INTERNATIONAL ORGANIZATIONS

OF THE

COMMITTEE ON FOREIGN AFFAIRS
HOUSE OF REPRESENTATIVES

ONE HUNDRED THIRTEENTH CONGRESS

SECOND SESSION

NOVEMBER 18, 2014

Serial No. 113–229

Printed for the use of the Committee on Foreign Affairs

Available via the World Wide Web: http://www.foreignaffairs.house.gov/ or http://www.gpo.gov/fdsys/

U.S. GOVERNMENT PRINTING OFFICE

91–452PDF   WASHINGTON : 2014

For sale by the Superintendent of Documents, U.S. Government Printing Office
Internet: bookstore.gpo.gov   Phone: toll free (866) 512–1800; DC area (202) 512–1800
Fax: (202) 512–2104   Mail: Stop IDCC, Washington, DC 20402–0001

(II)

CONTENTS

FIGHTING EBOLA: A GROUND–LEVEL VIEW

TUESDAY, NOVEMBER 18, 2014

House of Representatives,
Subcommittee on Africa, Global Health,
Global Human Rights, and International Organizations,
Committee on Foreign Affairs,
Washington, DC.

The subcommittee met, pursuant to notice, at 10:07 a.m., in room 2172, Rayburn House Office Building, Hon. Christopher H. Smith (chairman of the subcommittee) presiding.

Mr. SMITH. Subcommittee will come to order.

The world community has known of the Ebola virus disease, more commonly called just Ebola, since it first appeared in a remote region near the Democratic Republic of the Congo in 1976. In previous outbreaks, Ebola has been confined to remote areas in which there was little contact outside the villages at which it appeared.

Unfortunately, this outbreak, now an epidemic, spread from village to an international center for regional trade and spread into urban areas in Guinea, Sierra Leone, and Liberia that are crowded, with limited medical services and limited resident trust of government.

The unprecedented west African Ebola epidemic has not only killed more than 5,000 people with more than 14,000 others known to be affected, this situation has skewed the planning for how to deal with the outbreak.

In our two previous hearings on the Ebola epidemic, an emergency hearing we held on August 7 and then a followup on September 17, we heard about the worsening rates of infection and challenges in responding to this from government agencies, such as USAID and CDC, and NGOs operating on the ground, such as Samaritan's Purse and SIM.

Today's hearing is intended to take testimony from nongovernmental organizations providing services on the ground currently in the affected countries, especially Liberia, so we can better determine how proposed actions are being implemented.

In its early stages, Ebola manifests the same symptoms as less-immediately deadly diseases, such as malaria, which means initial healthcare workers have been unprepared for the deadly nature of the disease that they have been asked to treat.

This meant that too many healthcare workers, national and international, have been at risk in treating patients who themselves may not know they have Ebola. Hundreds of healthcare workers have been infected, and many have died, including some of top medical personnel in the three affected countries.

What we found quite quickly was that the healthcare systems in these countries, despite heavy investment by the United States and other donors, remained weak. As it happens, these are three countries either coming out of very divisive civil conflict or experiencing serious political divisions. Consequently, citizens have not been widely prepared to accept recommendations from their own governments.

For quite some time, many people in all three countries would not accept that the Ebola epidemic was real. Even now it is believed that, despite the prevalence of burial teams throughout Liberia, for example, some families are reluctant to identify their suffering and dead loved ones for safe burials, which places family members and their neighbors at heightened risk of contracting this often fatal disease when patients are most contagious.

The porous borders of these three countries have allowed people to cross between countries at will. This may facilitate commerce, which is a good thing, but it also allows for diseases to be transmitted regionally. As a result, the prevalence of Ebola in these three countries has ebbed and flowed with the migration of people from one country to the other.

Liberia remains the hardest hit of the three countries, with more than 6,500 Ebola cases officially recorded, probably a significant understatement. The number of infected and dead from Ebola could be as much as three times that of the official figure due to under-reporting.

Organizations operating on the ground have told us over the past 5 months that, despite the increasing reach of international and national efforts to contact those infected with Ebola, there remain many remote areas where it is still difficult to find residents or gain sufficient trust to obtain their cooperation.

Consequently, the ebb and flow in infection continues. Even when it looks like the battle is being won in one place, it increases in a neighboring country or region and then reignites in the areas that look to be successes.

The United States is focusing on Liberia. The UK is focusing on Sierra Leone. France and the European Union are supposed to be focusing on Guinea. In both Sierra Leone and Guinea, the anti-Ebola efforts are behind the pace of those in Liberia. This epidemic must be brought under control in all three if our efforts are to be successful.

Last week I, along with Congresswoman Karen Bass and Congressman Mark Meadows of this subcommittee, introduced H.R. 5710, the Ebola Emergency Response Act. This bill lays out steps that are needed for the U.S. Government to effectively help fight the west African Ebola epidemic, especially in Liberia, the worst hit of the three countries.

This includes recruiting and training healthcare personnel, establishing fully functional treatment centers, conducting education campaigns among populations in affected countries, and developing diagnostics, treatments, and vaccines.

H.R. 5710 confirms U.S. policy in the anti-Ebola fight and provides necessary authorities for the administration to continue or expand anticipated actions in this regard. The bill encourages U.S. collaboration with other donors to mitigate the risk of economic collapse and civil unrest in the three affected countries. Furthermore, the legislation authorizes funding of the International Disaster Assistance Account at the higher Fiscal Year 2014 level to effectively support these anti-Ebola efforts.

I would like to now turn to my friend and colleague, Ms. Bass, for any opening comments you might have.

Ms. BASS. As always, thank you, Chairman Smith, for your leadership and, also, for taking the lead on the legislation that we hope to have marked up soon.

I also want to thank today's distinguished witnesses and prominent NGO organizations providing critical medical, nutritional, and developmental assistance in the most adversely affected nations in west Africa.

I look forward to hearing your updates on how your respective organizations continue to combat this deadly outbreak, what trends you are seeing, both positive and negative, and what additional support is needed as you coordinate with the governments of the impacted countries in the international community.

I appreciate your efforts and outreach to help keep Congress informed of this evolving crisis. The current crisis, as has been stated, has been the largest and most widespread outbreak of the disease in history, creating a particular burden on the countries that are involved.

Since the beginning of the outbreak, U.S.-based NGOs have made a significant and sustained effort to support the three countries as they fought the disease. The United States has committed nearly $1 billion to build treatment centers, train healthcare workers and burial teams, supply hospitals with protective gear, and ensure the safety and humanitarian support.

I would, in particular, like to hear from the witnesses what you think about the assistance that has been provided. And then I have a particular interest in your thoughts around, when we are past this crisis, what the U.S. can leave in place and, also, your thoughts on how we move forward.

So we know that the reason why this hit so badly is because of the weak health infrastructure in these three countries.

So out of this terrible crisis, is there a way for us to begin to think long term about the future? How do we support the infrastructure of countries? And your thoughts on that would be appreciated.

The administration has asked Congress for over $6 billion in emergency funds in order to sustain the progress that has been made and to ensure an end to the crisis.

This request will expand assistance to contain the epidemic, safeguard the American public from further spread of the disease, and support the development of treatments. Sustained U.S. financial support and involvement is essential to support the stable governance of these nations, which is jeopardized by the current crisis.

I also don't think that we have given much time and attention to the fact that we are dealing with countries that could actually be moved quite a bit backward, especially countries that have recently gotten past civil war.

So I look forward to your testimonies, and I am interested in hearing from you about what we can do to assist your efforts.

Thank you.

Mr. SMITH. Thank you, Ms. Bass.

I'd like to now welcome our three very distinguished witnesses who are extraordinarily effective and informed and will provide this subcommittee a real insight as to what has been happening and what needs to be done.

Beginning with Mr. Rabih Torbay, who is the senior vice president for international operations and oversees International Medical Corps' global programs in 31 countries and 4 continents and its staff and volunteers numbering well over 8,000 people. He has personally supervised the expansion of IMC's humanitarian and development programs into some of the world's toughest working environments, including Sierra Leone, Iraq, Darfur, Liberia, Lebanon, Pakistan, Afghanistan, Haiti, Libya, and most recently Syria.

As the organization's senior representative in Washington, DC, he serves as IMC's liaison with the United States Government.

We will then hear from Mr. Brett Sedgewick, who is a technical advisor for food security and livelihoods for Global Communities. He previously served as vice president for the NASSCOM Foundation, for whom he built stakeholder relations with government entities, donors, and NGOs, and oversaw business development.

Prior to that, he served as Liberia country director for CHF International, where he oversaw program design, implementation, and monitoring for a range of donors. He also served as Liberia technical advisor to Chemonics on a similar basis.

We will then hear from Dr. Darius Mans, who is the president of Africare, where he is responsible for the leadership and growth of that organizations. Previously, he fulfilled a number of roles at the Millennium Challenge Corporation, including acting chief executive officer and vice president of implementation and managing director for Africare.

In these positions Dr. Mans was responsible for vast and diverse program portfolios in MCC compact countries. He also has experience managing 45 country programs around the world as director of the World Bank Institute, working as an economist, teaching economics, and serving as a consultant on infrastructure projects in Latin America.

We are joined by Mr. Weber, vice chairman of the subcommittee. Any opening comments?

Mr. WEBER. Thank you for being here. Let's go.

Mr. SMITH. Okay. Thank you.

I turn to Mr. Torbay.

STATEMENT OF MR. RABIH TORBAY, SENIOR VICE PRESIDENT FOR INTERNATIONAL OPERATIONS, INTERNATIONAL MEDICAL CORPS

Mr. TORBAY. Chairman Smith, Ranking Member Bass, and distinguished members of this subcommittee, on behalf of International Medical Corps, I would like to thank you for inviting me to testify today to describe the ongoing fight against the Ebola virus outbreak from the ground level.

I have already submitted a lengthy written testimony to the sub-committee. My remarks this morning will highlight key observations and offer 10 recommendations for our Ebola response experience.

International Medical Corps is a global humanitarian nonprofit organization dedicated to saving lives and relieving suffering through healthcare training and relief and development programs. We work in 31 countries around the world, and we have been working in west Africa since 1999.

Our response to the Ebola outbreak has been robust in both Liberia and Sierra Leone. More than two-thirds of all Ebola cases and over three-fourths of all Ebola-related deaths have come from these two countries.

By the end of this month, we anticipate having a total of about 800 staff in those two countries, and by year's end we expect this number to exceed 1,000 working in four Ebola treatment units, two in Liberia and two in Sierra Leone.

I would like to take this opportunity to acknowledge the dedicated and courageous international and African national staff working in our treatment centers. They are from Liberia and Sierra Leone, as well as many parts of the United States, Europe, and other states.

Our staff is comprised of doctors, nurses, technicians, specialists in water sanitation and hygiene, logisticians, mental health professionals, custodial workers, and burial teams.

In addition to the treatment units, we have established several services for groups just now arriving to combat the outbreak. One example is a training center on the ground of Cuttington University in Bong County, Liberia. It will teach and train staff from all organizations engaged in the fight to contain Ebola and show them how to treat patients and stay safe in a potentially dangerous workplace.

We are also responding to the upsurge of Ebola cases in Mali. We will be setting up an Ebola treatment unit and developing a health worker training program to help the country fight the outbreak.

Our robust response to the Ebola outbreak has one overriding objective: Contain the current outbreak at its source in west Africa. To succeed, we have learned that several key factors must be in place.

One of these is building and safely operating Ebola treatment units staffed by well-trained health professionals. Another key factor is using training programs to transfer into local hands the skills and knowledge necessary to respond effectively to the Ebola outbreaks.

We must also assure effective coordination among all actors involved in the fight to contain the virus, including the U.N., international and national governments, and NGOs. To turn the tide of this epidemic, we must all work together to maximize the strength of all involved.

Finally, we need to conduct expansive data collection and rigorous data analysis to build an accurate picture of Ebola containment and spot any need for new responses. Once we succeed to contain the current outbreak, we must remain vigilant to assure that there is no resurgence of this epidemic.

The fight to contain Ebola and prevent future outbreaks will require a substantial investment. I would like to thank the U.S. Agency for International Development, particularly its Office of Foreign Disaster Assistance, for the funding it has provided to International Medical Corps for our Ebola response, as well as the support of the U.S. military, particularly in setting up a laboratory near in our Ebola treatment unit in Bong County.

We welcome the President's emergency request to Congress to combat Ebola in west Africa. And based on our on-the-ground experience in fighting this epidemic, we would recommend that the $1.4 billion allocated for international disaster assistance be increased by an additional $200 million, to a total of $1.6 billion, and we recommend that an additional $48 million be added to the Economic Support Fund, for a total of $260 million.

Mr. Chairman, I conclude my testimony by offering 10 recommendations for effective treatment and eradication of Ebola virus for the subcommittee's consideration.

One, ensure the availability of an adequate number of well-trained, well-protected health workers. One of the most critical lessons learned from this response has been the importance of having sufficient human resources prepared to address an outbreak of infectious disease.

Two, ensure that construction of new Ebola treatment units fits the local needs. The work must be well-coordinated and well-trained staff must be ready to work in each facility. We need to remain flexible and nimble and adapt quickly to changing demands to response to outbreaks in rural areas.

Three, ensure that the necessary quantity and quality of personal protective equipment is available.

Four, improve data collection, surveillance, and referral systems that will help individuals receive treatment faster.

Five, ensure that clear and understandable lines of communications and divisions of responsibilities are established, understood, and maintained among coordinating bodies operating in the region. A smart and efficient coordination system at the national level is critical for an effective response.

Six, we welcome the advances made over the past few weeks in establishing procedure to evacuate and treat expatriate health workers who might contract Ebola. We recommend that the systems being put in place now be institutionalized and made part of the global preparedness planning in the future for future epidemics.

Seven, we recommend that commercial airspace over Ebola countries remain open so that personnel and resources can move quickly.

Eight, accelerate and support the production of vaccines.

Nine, invest in emergency preparedness in west African regions to ensure that these countries have the needed resources, proper training, and systems in place to respond themselves to possible future outbreak of infectious disease.

And, ten, finally, Mr. Chairman, basic health services need to be re-established in west Africa. People are not just dying from Ebola, they are dying from malaria, they are dying from water-borne diseases. Women are dying from the lack of facilities where they could go for safe delivery. And this needs to be done as soon as possible. We cannot wait until the Ebola outbreak is done before we restart these activities.

Thank you, Mr. Chairman and Ranking Member Bass, for the opportunity to present this testimony to the committee. I would be glad to answer any questions you may have.

[The prepared statement of Mr. Torbay follows:]

Statement of Mr. Rabih Torbay

Senior Vice President for International Operations

International Medical Corps

Before the

Subcommittee on Africa, Global Health, Global Human Rights

& International Organizations

Of the House Committee on Foreign Affairs

"Fighting Ebola: A Ground Level View"

Nov. 18, 2014

Chairman Smith, Ranking Member Bass and distinguished members of the subcommittee. On behalf of International Medical Corps, one of only a small handful of international NGOs treating Ebola patients in West Africa, I would like to thank you for inviting me to testify today. My statement addresses the emergency response to the Ebola virus epidemic in West Africa and the status of health conditions at the ground level.

International Medical Corps is a global, humanitarian, nonprofit organization dedicated to saving lives and relieving suffering through health care training and relief and development programs. Its mission is to improve the quality of life through health interventions and related activities that build local capacity in underserved communities worldwide. By offering training and health care to local populations and medical assistance to people at highest risk, and with the flexibility to respond rapidly to emergency situations, International Medical Corps rehabilitates broken health care systems and helps restore them to self-reliance.

My remarks today will largely be confined to our operations in Liberia and Sierra Leone—where more than two-thirds of all Ebola cases and over three-quarters of all Ebola-related deaths have been reported. I will also refer briefly to conditions in Mali, where we are seeing an upsurge of infections.

Our response to the Ebola outbreak has been robust. By the end of this month we anticipate having a total staff of about 800 in Liberia and Sierra Leone, of which 90 percent are African nationals. By year's end we expect this number to reach 1,000 working in four Ebola Treatment Units in Liberia and Sierra Leone.

When the first Ebola cases were detected in the region in late 2013, International Medical Corps was already operational in Sierra Leone, providing community level health care, mental health care, and support in the fight against malnutrition. Given International Medical Corps longstanding work and familiarity with the West Africa region, where we have operated health and humanitarian assistance programs since 1999, we learned of the Ebola outbreak almost immediately, and monitored the pace of the disease closely.

Between mid-June and mid-July, the number of confirmed cases of Ebola in Sierra Leone grew from fewer than 20 per week to more than 50. During the second half of July, the number of confirmed cases reported in Liberia also increased. After immediate discussions with our field teams and also with partner agencies to assess needs and gaps, we realized the epidemic was moving out of control.

By this time, we had already deployed teams to Sierra Leone to work with local NGOs as part of a community-level campaign to raise awareness about Ebola. The day after Sierra Leone President Ernest Bai Koroma declared a state of emergency, August 1st, we ordered a rapid assessment of local conditions and triggered our highest category of emergency response. We also determined the more urgent task was no longer raising public awareness but treating those who had contracted the virus. Our Emergency Response Team arrived in Sierra Leone soon after and since then has worked vigorously to contain the epidemic .

In Liberia, we employed our highest category of emergency response and ordered a rapid assessment of conditions in early August. Our Emergency Response Team arrived in Monrovia 72 hours after Liberian President Ellen Johnson declared a state of national emergency in the country. What our team found on the ground in Liberia confirmed that urgent action was required. In a few short months, fallout from the Ebola outbreak had brought the country's already fragile health care system to the brink of collapse. Previously busy hospitals and clinics were empty, with both staff and potential patients too frightened seek treatment for routine health issues for fear of being infected with the virus. Rather than risk infection, mothers shunned life-saving vaccinations for their children, and if their child became ill, all too many believed the safer option was to not seek treatment at all.

For International Medical Corps, coordination in emergency response is crucial to success. In these critical circumstances, we reached out to key actors, such as the World Health Organization (WHO), the Centers for Disease Control and Prevention (CDC), and USAID even before we deployed our own teams. Once on the ground in Liberia, we immediately began coordinating our work with other groups responding to the Ebola crisis, particularly Liberia's

Ministry of Health and Social Welfare, as well as representatives of USAID's Disaster Assistance Response Team (DART), WHO, the CDC and. other NGOs.

As part of an Incident Management System established to tackle the Ebola outbreak, International Medical Corps quickly agreed to manage and provide the necessary staff for an Ebola Treatment Unit (ETU) built by Save the Children in the Suakoko District of Bong County, about a four-hour drive north of the capital, Monrovia. Médecins Sans Frontières (MSF) graciously trained our key staff who would be operating the ETU. The Ministry of Health provided us with a cadre of national health workers that would staff the ETU and the management of Cuttington University provided their dormitories to house our staff, as well as other administrative buildings. We are thankful to all for their support.

We admitted our first patients to the Bong County ETU on September 15th. Currently, the facility is staffed by a team of 17 expatriates and 161 Liberian nationals. We are gradually building up to 70 beds and a staff of around 230, of which 90 percent are African nationals. As of Nov. 14, the Bong County ETU had admitted 279 patients. To date, 73 patients have died, 134 patients suspected of having Ebola have been discharged after tests for the disease came back negative, and 34 are currently receiving care (26 confirmed, 11 suspected cases awaiting lab tests). A total of 36 patients have been discharged as recovered.

I would like to acknowledge the dedicated and courageous international and African national staff working in our treatment centers. They have come from inside Liberia and outside – including physicians and nurses from many parts of the United States, Europe and Africa. Our staff is comprised of doctors, nurses, technicians, specialists in water, sanitation and hygiene, logisticians, mental health professionals, custodial workers, and members of burial teams.

To date, our Bong County ETU remains one of just two in Liberia operating outside of Monrovia. Our operations there involve isolating and treating patients, providing them with counseling, caring for the remains of those who succumb to the disease and operating an ambulance service dedicated to transporting suspected Ebola patients to the ETU and returning those home who have either recovered or tested negatively for the virus. We are also assisting in the reintegration of those returnees to communities that may be anxious about their return, and working with local NGOs on patient referrals.

After discussions with the Ministry of Health, WHO, the CDC, DART and the U.S. military, the U.S. Navy established a laboratory at Cuttington University, adjacent to our Bong County ETU. The presence of this laboratory and its ability to turn around the results of blood test for Ebola quickly has made a major difference to our work. It has also saved many lives by allowing those who test negative for the disease to leave the ETU far sooner than previously—cutting the wait time for results from as long as five days to a matter of 5-7 hours. I want to take this opportunity to express my personal thanks to the U.S. military for establishing the laboratory in Bong.

International Medical Corps anticipates opening a second ETU with 100 beds in Kakata, Margibi County, which borders Bong County to the southwest, by the end of November.

In Liberia, International Medical Corps will also establish mobile technical support units comprised of Ebola clinical specialists as well as experts in mental health and psycho-social support, logistics, site management and water, sanitation and hygiene. These units will deploy to partners' sites, providing them ongoing training, guidance and start-up assistance as they establish their own ETUs in the country. .

In addition, International Medical Corps will maintain an urgent-response team of skilled senior staff (both expatriate and national) that can deploy quickly to fill short-term gaps should an ETU have urgent staffing needs. International Medical Corps will also be operating an ambulance dedicated solely fto transport health workers who become infected to the United States Public Health Service-run Mobile Medical Unit from anywhere outside of Monrovia. The ambulance would be staffed by our trained ambulance teams.

In Sierra Leone we are preparing to open a 50-bed Ebola Treatment Unit in Lunsar on Nov. 25, and a 100-bed ETU in Makeni on Dec. 11. They are funded by USAID and the British government. A laboratory will also be built in Makeni. The ETUs will ensure that health care providers (doctors, nurses, community health workers, midwives, and traditional birth attendants) and water, sanitation and hygiene specialists, are formally trained on infection control protocols, EVD case management, and/or PPE usage. International Medical Corps will also be managing and supervising two to four 10-bed screening and referral units (SRU) to ensure optimal patient care and infection control.

On November 8, International Medical Corps opened a training center, located on the grounds of Cuttington University in Bong Country, Liberia, to train staff of international and national organizations who will be treating Ebola patients. Physicians and nurses coming into direct contact with Ebola patients will receive up to 12 days training, while other essential skilled technical staff, such as logisticians and water and sanitation engineers, will receive 7-10 days. Among those we are training are members of a U.S. Public Health Service team who will staff a 25-bed Ebola Treatment Unit in Monrovia dedicated to treating health workers who have been infected with the disease during the course of their work treating others. A similar training center will be established in Sierra Leone before the end of the year.

Such hands-on training is the key to protecting health workers who must operate in an environment where all know the Ebola virus is present. Strong guidelines and regulations are important, but they must be combined with hands-on training to be truly effective.

In Mali, together with Plan International, we are developing a training program to help prepare that country to respond to an Ebola outbreak. Discussions are underway to establish a training center in Bamako that will provide didactic and practical training for health care professionals and community members working in the areas of infection control, contact tracing and case management. We project the training program will begin by the end of November.

Procedures, Protocols and Practice

In its 30 years of providing humanitarian assistance to those in need, International Medical Corps has worked in more than 70 countries in some of the world's toughest, most dangerous environments, but had not previously encountered the Ebola virus or treated patients infected with it. However, our experience of working consistently in challenging, high-risk conditions taught us to move carefully, expect the unexpected and to err on the side of caution when weighing risk as we prepared to open our first treatment unit. We consulted with staff from Médecins Sans Frontières to draw on the depth of their experience and the guidelines and protocols they had developed in treating Ebola patients during previous outbreaks in Africa. We also reviewed guidelines and protocols from the CDC and WHO.

We learned quickly that treating Ebola patients is a labor-intensive endeavor that demands exceptionally strong logistics to maintain the flow of large quantities of supplies, including personal protective equipment (PPE) for the staff, bedding and medications for patients, as well as disinfectant and water to keep the treatment unit safe and clean. For example, most PPEs can be used only once, then are incinerated to prevent possible infection. We require approximately 840 PPEs per week per ETU to comply with guidelines established to ensure the safety of our staff. We follow a ratio using 3 expatriate doctors per 50 patients, 8 expatriate nurses per 50 patients, 4 local physician assistants per 50 patients, 24 local nurses per 50 patients, and 2 consumable PPEs per patient.

To treat Ebola patients effectively, we require a staff of about 230 to operate a 70-bed treatment unit. This is a staff per patient ratio of over 3:1. Ebola treatment requires higher than normal staff levels to reduce the risk of mistakes that could potentially endanger both patients and staff. One common practice in our ETUs is for members of our teams to work in pairs — what we call a "buddy system." For example, two physicians or two nurses make every decision that in a regular setting would be made by one on their own. Each "buddy" is constantly checking the personal protective equipment of the other and that the delivery of care is running correctly. The "buddy system" is also used when removing a PPE, a procedure that can carry a high risk of infection if not done properly. To further diminish risk, we have also added one more Shift Supervisor, whose task is to make sure each "buddy team" is following the prescribed protocols and to monitor the overall movement of the team and the treatment it is delivering to our patients. Our staff follow very specific and meticulous, step-by-step donning and doffing protocols.

These protocols are demanding and arduous, requiring personal discipline, concentration and patience on the part of all involved. They are needed because the danger to staff can be very high. We are painfully aware that as of middle of this month, more than 560 health workers had been infected with Ebola in the course of their work. Of these, 320 have died. In Liberia, Ebola has been nicknamed "the nurse killer".

I am pleased to report the strict guidelines and protocols we have implemented have been successful. We have been able to both protect and treat health workers at the Bong facility. Actually, one of the patients we admitted and treated was a Liberian nurse infected while caring for Ebola patients at another facility. She has recovered and is now working at our ETU.

Our protocols require that PPEs worn by our staff cover the entire body. No skin can show. We quickly learned that wearing a bulky, impermeable PPE with as many as three layers of protection in West Africa's high humidity with temperatures of 95 degrees means that staff can only work relatively short periods of time—usually between 1 and 2 hours maximum—inside the unit's restricted area before being rotated and replaced by another team.

In addition to the ETUs, a new approach is to be implemented in Liberia and Sierra Leone that we believe will help contain the Ebola virus. Community Care Centers are being established enabling suspected Ebola patients to be removed from their homes and relocated inta community-based center where they could be isolated and provided with palliative care without the danger of infecting family and other potential care-givers in the home. Each Community Care Center would have approximately 10 beds where patients could await testing. A patient testing positive for Ebola could be transferred to an ETU for treatment while those who test negative would be allowed to return home. We would support this concept as long as the health workers serving in such centers receive both full training and are equipped with the same PPEs as those used in ETUs. The centers should also need to be linked to—and supported by—an ETU, acting as de facto satellites to that ETU.

Funding, Needs and Support

We are grateful for the timely and generous funding we have received from USAID's Office of Foreign Disaster Assistance (OFDA), which enabled us to open our first ETU in Bong County and to prepare our staff training facility nearby. OFDA also funded the ETU nearing completion in Lunsar, Sierra Leone. Other government donors have come forward as well to address the crisis, as have some private foundations and corporations. However, generating public donations, which are necessary to support our efforts to fight Ebola, has been a challenge.

As we continue to increase our presence in both Liberia and Sierra Leone for what we believe will be a prolonged fight to contain the Ebola virus in West Africa, our needs will grow accordingly. Put simply, we need three things: people, commodities, and money. We need to continue the recruitment and training of staff and to build a "human resources" pipeline. Conditions to facilitate this—which include travel to and from the affected countries, procedures and systems to protect and treat health workers—must be ensured and implemented as soon as possible.

By commodities, I mean everything from PPEs to disinfectant, to vehicles for transportation, mattresses and bed clothing. Many of these items can only be used once because of the need to contain the spread of the disease.

The fight to contain Ebola and prevent future outbreaks will require a substantial investment. While we welcome the president's emergency request to Congress to combat Ebola in West Africa, based on our experience in fighting this disease on the ground, we would recommend that the $1.4 billion allocated for International Disaster Assistance be increased by $200 million to $1.6 billion. We recommend that an additional $48 million be added to the Economic Support Fund for a total of $260 million. The math is pretty basic: assuming there are 27 ETUs regionally, and 120 Community Care Centers, we anticipate it would require about $1.6 billion for the next 6 months to bring the disease under control. We will also need to consider the secondary impact of the outbreak—the added costs of food, security, and loss of economic activity are estimated at $500 million. Rebuilding the health care system and maintaining an adequate disease surveillance system could run an additional $600 million.

What Works

Mr. Chairman, I would now like to briefly share some of our lessons learned of what we know works. I believe this will help highlight several key areas of focus as we move forward.

First and foremost, we need to contain the disease at its source in west Africa. For that to happen, we have learned several factors must be in place. One of these includes having operational ETUs staffed by well-trained health professionals.

Community Care Centers, if well-staffed and equipped, could help limit the transmission. A robust referral system between the care centers and ETUs, as well as between ETUs could take advantage of available bed capacity that now exist in some facilities and alleviate pressure of other ETUs that are overloaded. This can help reduce the wait, time, transmission rate and mortality rates. Limiting the spread of the virus in the community is essential to the containment plan. Therefore, a focus on community sensitization, including education, awareness and outreach to build a trusting environment is of utmost important.

Second, building local capacity by carrying out training and supervision of local personnel provides countries with the needed tools and mechanisms to to respond on their own during outbreaks. The approach to this should be comprehensive and include the various components that are essential to containing, preventing and treating Ebola—from infection control and prevention, contact tracing, case management and treatment, to safe burial.

Third, we must focus on strengthening coordination of all actors – the UN, internationaland national governments and NGOs. To turn the tide of this epidemic, we need to work together and use the strengths of all stakeholders involved.

Fourth, expansive data collection and rigorous data analysis are essential in order to build an accurate picture of Ebola containment and spot any need for new responses. This information must be shared among all involved in a timely manner.

What is Needed Going Forward

As we have stated above when describing our response, the most critical challenge is addressing the scarcity of health workers needed to treat patients and staff ETUs that are currently in operation and those now being planned and built.

We face a severe shortage of adequately trained health professionals, both national and international. The difficult work environment, the personal risk, the need for 21 day self-isolation in some circumstances, all make it difficult for us to recruit volunteers. Health care workers also want to be assured that there are clear plans and procedures in place for possible evacuation and treatment should they fall ill. This has been slow in coming. The growing restrictions on travel to and from West Africa will only isolate the affected countries further, compromise the supply chain and inhibit efforts to recruit qualified staff. These factors will further enable the severe outbreak to continue.

Once recruited, the training of health workers and first responders continues to be a major need. This includes training of staff working in a treatment units, at community care centers, and on burial teams. It also includes ambulance attendants, community workers and educators. The training being conducted by the CDC, the training to be conducted by the U.S. military, training being led by NGOs, including International Medical Corps must be supported. We, at International Medical Corps, are willing to train ETU staff, both in Sierra Leone and Liberia, to help contain the virus.

I would also like to underscore how vital the availability and proper use of PPEs has been—and continues to be— during the Ebola response. It is important to note that acquiring appropriate personal protective equipment has been a significant challenge given the the limited number of available qualified suppliers and the large volume of PPEs required to staff treatment centers at effective levels . . The current demand far exceeds the supply. We need to talk about the need for more accurate data, the need to review our plans constantly, be flexible, nimble and adaptable

Mr. Chairman, I conclude my testimony with ten recommendations for the Committee's consideration.

1. Ensure the availability of adequate, well-trained, well-protected health workers. One of the most critical lessons learned from this response has been the importance of having the human resources ready and prepared to address an outbreak of infectious disease. Cadres of health workers and community members need to be well-trained (and supported) to staff the treatment units and care centers in the affected countries and carry out other components of the response such as safe burials, contact tracing and social mobilization. This is critical not only for the immediate response but also to prepare other countries in the region for any potential future outbreaks and ensure that they have skilled personnel in place to be able to respond on their own. To be truly effective, it is important that the training of personnel be led by organizations with hands-on experience in treatment and management of Ebola cases and that it involve actual practical training with personal protective equipment and mock patients and not be limited to classroom study and power point presentations.

2. Ensure that the construction of new ETUs fits the needs of each country. The work must be well coordinated and well-trained staff ready to work in each facility. Flexible and reactive staffing models are necessary to respond to outbreaks in rural areas. Patient transport outside of Monrovia must be improved, including deployment of more ambulances, training of teams, and establishment of strong dispatch and coordination systems.

3. Ensure that the necessary quantity and quality of Personal Protective Equipment (PPE) is available.

4. Improve data collection, surveillance and referral systems that will help individuals receive treatment quickly and strengthen the link between community-based and referral-systems.

5. Establish clear and understandable linkages among coordinating bodies that are now in place, including the UN Mission for Ebola Emergency Response and country coordination bodies. Ensure that all operational groups are connected to these

coordination mechanisms. A smart and efficient coordination mechanism at the national level is critical for effectiveness of the response.

6. While we welcome the advances made over the past few weeks in establishing procedures to evacuate and treat expatriate health workers who might contract Ebola, we recommend that the systems being put in place now be institutionalized and made part of the global preparedness planning in the event of future epidemics. ETU-caliber staff should be employed at primary health facilities and a capable ambulance network should be created to move people to ETUs as quickly possible if they meet the case definition.

7. Maintain open commercial airspace over Ebola-affected countries so that personnel and resources can be moved quickly.

8. Accelerate and support the production of vaccines.

9. Invest in health preparedness in the West Africa region to ensure these countries have the needed resources, proper training and systems in place to respond themselves to possible future outbreaks of infectious diseases.

10. Revive health care services that have been affected so dramatically by the outbreak. Some of the most serious side effects of the Ebola outbreak occurred when basic health care delivery systems failed nationally. As a result, Sierra Leone and Liberia, which have already experienced some of the highest levels of maternal and child deaths, now face conditions where there are no available facilities for women to have C-sections or children to be immunized. There are no trauma centers to treat accident victims or facilities to continue to manage ongoing severe health problems affecting the local populations including high rates of malaria, pneumonia, and a wide range of chronic conditions. As a result, the mortality rate is expected to increase to higher levels. A vigorous effort must be made to restore access to primary and secondary health services as quickly as possible. Building stronger health care systems as part of recovery and long-term health strategy in the region is critical.

Thank you Mr. Chairman and Ranking Member Bass for the opportunity to present this testimony to the committee. I would be glad to answer any questions.

Mr. SMITH. Thank you very much, Mr. Torbay.

Mr. Sedgewick, if you could proceed.

STATEMENT OF MR. BRETT SEDGEWICK, TECHNICAL ADVISOR FOR FOOD SECURITY AND LIVELIHOODS, GLOBAL COMMUNITIES

Mr. SEDGEWICK. Chairman Smith, Ranking Member Bass, members of the subcommittee, thank you for the opportunity to testify today on the ways we are working to stop the Ebola epidemic in west Africa.

The following is an abbreviated version of the written testimony provided to the subcommittee.

My name is Brett Sedgewick, and I am technical advisor at Global Communities, formerly known as CHF International, and I am currently on the Ebola Task Force.

From 2010 to 2011, I worked as Global Communities' Liberia country director, and I returned to the U.S. 10 days ago after spending 3 weeks in Liberia helping to lead our response on the ground.

Global Communities has worked in Liberia since 2004. In 2010, we began a USAID-funded water and sanitation project, working closely with the Ministry of Health and Social Welfare. Through this program, we began to combat Ebola in April by providing community education, protective equipment, and hygiene materials to communities at risk.

In August, we partnered with USAID's Office of Foreign Disaster Assistance, who have been excellent partners in this fight, to scale up our response. Today we are also working in safe burial and body management, contact tracing, and ambulance services.

Safe body management is of the highest priority in stopping the spread of Ebola. The bodies of Ebola victims are extremely contagious. In Liberia, it is often customary for the family of the deceased to say goodbye through traditions that involve touching and washing the body. The CDC estimates that up to 70 percent of Ebola infections are originating from contact with the deceased.

Global Communities is working in every county of Liberia, supporting 47 burial teams and 32 disinfection teams. We work in close partnership with the Ministry of Health. The ministry employ the burial team personnel, and we provide training, vehicles, logistical support, and equipment.

The work of burial teams is both backbreaking and heartbreaking. I have accompanied burial teams and seen the incredible professionalism with which they operate. These men and women work covered in impermeable materials in high temperatures, hiking hours through thick jungle, taking canoes or assembling makeshift bridges over bodies of water.

They enter communities stricken with grief and fear and carry out an incredibly sensitive task with the greatest care for their health and for that of others. These men and women are heroes of this crisis that deserve our gratitude for assuming great risk and social isolation in order to stop this epidemic. While risky, this work can be done safely. Not one of our more than 500 team members have contracted the virus.

This work is not without challenges. Many resist identifying their dead as infected. They fear they will not be able to mourn their loved ones and they themselves will be stigmatized. This is why the work of safe burial goes hand in hand with community engagement. Many burial rites are safe, and the teams let communities safely and respectfully say goodbye to their loved ones.

Another challenge is cremation. In Montserrado County, which contains Monrovia, cremation became official policy during the height of the outbreak. However, this practice is counter to traditional practices and is met with strong resistance.

The idea of a deceased loved one being burned, in their vernacular, upset many and increased stigma and contributes to bodies being unsafely buried or the sick being hidden.

To combat this, Global Communities, USAID, and the Liberian Government are exploring safe burials in Montserrado through identifying land that can accommodate a large number of burials and has space for families to safely gather and mourn.

Despite the challenges, safe burial is proving highly effective. We began burial team support in August for Bong, Lofa, and Nimba Counties. By the first week of October, we had expanded to support teams in every county of Liberia. And last month they were able to collect 96 percent of bodies within 24 hours.

We were also able to directly reach over 1,500 communities through meeting and dialogue sessions, bringing together senior government officials, county health teams, traditional chiefs, religious leaders, community health volunteers, and other local leaders.

Indeed, it is now being widely reported that we are seeing the rate of infection slow throughout Liberia, which is cause for optimism. However, it is not yet time for celebration. We must maintain the level of vigilance that has proven effective and beginning to control the spread of the virus. Significant longer term investments must be made in the health systems of the country.

In closing, Global Communities would like to express profound gratitude for Congress, particularly members of this committee, for your continued support of this work. The worst Ebola outbreak in history can be stopped and will be stopped.

I look forward to your questions.

[The prepared statement of Mr. Sedgewick follows:]

"Fighting Ebola: A Ground-Level View"

Testimony by
Brett Sedgewick
Technical Advisor, Ebola Taskforce, Global Communities

Before the
House Foreign Affairs Committee
Subcommittee on Africa, Global Health, and Global Human Rights,
and International Organizations
November 18, 2014

Chairman Smith, Ranking Member Bass, members of the committee, thank you for the opportunity to testify before you today on ways we are working to stop the epidemic of Ebola in West Africa.

My name is Brett Sedgewick and I work as Technical Advisor to the Ebola Taskforce at Global Communities. From 2010 to 2011 I worked for Global Communities as the Liberia Country Director. I returned to the United States 10 days ago, after spending three weeks in Liberia, helping to lead our response against Ebola on the ground.

Global Communities has partnered with communities in Liberia since 2004, immediately after the end of the Liberian civil war. We began by working to bring communities together through peacebuilding and reconciliation. In the decade since, we have invested in the counties of Lofa, Bong, and Nimba, as well as Monrovia, building strong partnerships with the traditional leaders of these counties and with government entities at the national and county levels. In 2010, we began to implement the five-year, USAID-funded Improved Water, Sanitation and Hygiene program (IWASH) that focuses on the Community Led Total Sanitation methodology. We worked closely with the Ministry of Health and Social Welfare to empower communities to improve their overall health primarily through better hygiene practices, buttressed by improved water supply systems and sanitation facilities.

Global Communities began combating the spread of Ebola in April by providing community education, protective equipment and hygiene materials to communities through our existing program with USAID. This summer, as the Ebola outbreak spread, we partnered with USAID's Office of Foreign Disaster Assistance (OFDA) to further leverage our community and government partnerships in order to combat the spread of the disease. Our activities aim to combat infection through community engagement and education, safe burial and body management, contact tracing, and ambulance services. While my esteemed co-witnesses here are working to save those are ill, we are complementing these efforts by focusing on saving those who are well from being infected by those we have lost.

Throughout the epidemic, Liberia has been the hardest hit of the affected countries, and the scale of disaster has been overwhelming. Beyond the immediate health effects, we are seeing second-tier effects of the outbreak: economic downturn, food insecurity, unemployment, a huge number of orphans and child head of households, and potential instability. All this in a country that was already among the least developed nations in the world, but was facing its challenges and overcoming them. We must make every effort to stop both the disease and the deleterious effects it is leaving behind in its wake.

Due to the nature of how Ebola is transmitted, at Global Communities we have focused our immediate and greatest efforts on safe burial and body management. Ebola is spread through bodily fluids that increase in their level of contagion as the virus multiplies throughout the body and the patient becomes increasingly ill. Those most at risk for contracting the virus are those caring for the sick, and those handling the dead. As the viral load is the typically highest at the moment of death, a person who has recently passed away is extremely contagious. In the case of Liberia, it is customary for the family of the deceased to say goodbye through traditions that involve touching and washing of the body. This is one of the primary ways that Ebola gained so strong a foothold in Liberia, particularly in Monrovia where the high population density reinforced the rapid spread. The CDC estimates that before safe burial practices began to be implemented, up to 70 percent of cases were originating from contact with the deceased. Consequently, safe body management is of the highest priority in stopping the spread of Ebola.

Through our partnership with USAID OFDA, which is to be commended for the speed and skill with which it is responding, Global Communities is currently supporting 47 burial teams and 32 disinfection teams active throughout all 15 counties of Liberia. This approach is complemented by community education and engagement which enables every aspect of safe body management to be based on community feedback. Global Communities provides training, vehicles, logistical support, and equipment to the burial teams. This would not be possible without very close partnership with the Liberian Ministry of Health and Social Welfare (MoHSW). It was our existing relationship with this ministry that enabled us to scale up our work so quickly. The networks, resources, and trust needed to successfully engage in safe body management and community engagement were already in place. This partnership also ensures that the face of the response is Liberian, that we learn from what works and what does not, and that the capacity of the Ministry is being strengthened as it responds to the needs of the crisis. It is a common misconception that the MoHSW has been devastated by this crisis. While clinical infrastructure certainly has been severely damaged, other parts of the Ministry, such as the Environmental Health Technicians, have been trained and empowered.

Most importantly, the MoHSW employs the personnel that make up the burial teams. A burial team consists of a team lead, usually a county-level environmental health technician, two drivers, four carriers, and two chlorine sprayers. Once the county health team receives a call that a body has been identified, the team mobilizes and travels to the body, often in remote areas that require complicated logistics to access. Once in position, every member of the team dons personal protective equipment according to CDC and WHO guidelines. The team then approaches the body which is heavily sprayed with chlorine along with the surrounding area and materials. The body is sealed in a body bag and then transported to the gravesite. Once the body is in the grave, the team carefully removes all protective equipment and places it into the grave to be buried along with the body. The grave is filled in, sprayed again, and then each team member is sprayed and decontaminated as is the vehicle.

The work is hard, backbreaking and often heartbreaking. I have accompanied burial teams and seen the incredible professionalism and care with which they operate. The team members work while covered in impermeable materials in very high temperatures, often hiking through thick jungle, taking boats or assembling make-shift bridges over bodies of water. They enter communities stricken with grief and fear and carry out an incredibly sensitive task. These men and women are heroes of this crisis that deserve our recognition and gratitude for assuming great personal risk in order to stop this epidemic. While risky, however, burial and body management can be done safely when done correctly. To date, not one of our team members has contracted the virus. That is more than 500 people safely engaged in an extremely dangerous profession. Ebola can be managed and controlled.

However, burial team and body management is not without its challenges. In Liberia, the Ebola virus is shrouded in stigma and many families resist identifying their dead as having the virus. They fear they will not have the chance to mourn their loved one and that they themselves will be stigmatized and ostracized. This is why the work of safe burial goes hand in hand with community education and engagement. Education about the virus reduces fear and stigma, and engagement and relationship building increase trust, respect, and cultural sensitivity. Our burial teams approach communities with a mindset of engagement and partnership. Burials are done safely, but allow family and friends to participate as much as possible. While not all burial rites are safe, many are, and allowing communities to respectfully say goodbye to their loved ones ensures that they will invite us in the next time someone passes.

The response also requires a huge amount of flexibility and adaptation. Our activities have been customized by county based on what we've experienced on the ground. We have had to create new types of teams on the fly, like walking teams and canoe teams, which are able to reach some of the most remote communities in the world.

Another challenge we have encountered is opposition to cremation. In Monsterrado County, the area surrounding Monrovia, cremation is being practiced due to the high population density of the area and the high Ebola caseload. However, this has met with strong resistance. The idea of taking a sick loved one to a treatment center then never seeing them again and learning that they were "burned" (in their vernacular) was found unacceptable and soundly rejected at the community level. This increased stigma and contributed to bodies unsafely buried and the sick not being sent to Ebola Treatment Units. Again, the answer has been to work in partnership with communities to develop a culturally appropriate solution. Global Communities, USAID and the Liberian government are currently exploring safe burials in Montserrado County through securing appropriate land to be developed into a cemetery that can not only accommodate a large number of bodies but which also has space for families to safely gather and mourn.

Despite the challenges, safe burial is proving effective in stopping the spread of Ebola. Global Communities began burial team support in August. Since then, despite these challenges, we have been able to collect an average of 93 percent of all bodies within 24 hours of death. By the first week of October, we had burial teams in every country of Liberia and last month our teams were able to collect 96 percent of bodies within 24 hours.

Community education makes this possible, and is also working, making communities more aware of the precautions they must take to keep themselves safe and healthy. In Lofa County, a hotbed of the virus in the beginning of the outbreak, communities are taking ownership of their health by physically fencing themselves in, monitoring travel, and being vigilant about safe burial. They have also developed a triage system that allows them to identify Ebola versus other illnesses and take appropriate steps to keep the uninfected safe. As a result, Lofa County has seen the numbers of Ebola cases drop significantly, and saw zero cases for several weeks in October. Across Liberia, we were able to directly reach over 1,500 communities in some of the critically important areas of the response through Community Meeting and Dialogue Sessions. These meetings bring together senior members of the Ministry of Health and Social Welfare with traditional chiefs, religious leaders, town criers, community health volunteers, and other local leaders.

Indeed, it has now been widely reported that we are seeing the caseload slow in growth throughout Liberia, which is cause for optimism. However, it is not yet time for celebration or to let our guard down. The international community, the government of Liberia, and the people of Liberia themselves must maintain the level of vigilance and the behavior change that has proven effective in beginning to control the spread of the virus, and stay the course until the epidemic is halted. Community education must also continue so the people of Liberia are empowered to maintain their own health. Significant, longer-term investments must be made in the health systems of the country, particularly in the capacity of the Ministry of Health and Social Welfare which is critically important to preventing other outbreaks of disease in the future. Ensuring their ability to respond now will leave behind a strong and dedicated environmental health system for the future. We all must learn from this outbreak to prevent future such disasters.

Even when the epidemic appears to be safely under control, we will still need to remain cautious, attentive, and responsive. Global Communities has seen through its work in other post-conflict and disaster settings around the world that there is often a dangerous gap between emergency response and long-term investment. Areas such as food security and economic stability can often suffer during this time frame. Investing in those areas now will prevent additional setbacks in the future. Remaining attentive will also ensure that there will not be a period where Ebola is allowed to thrive again.

In closing, Global Communities would like to express profound gratitude to Congress, particularly the members of this committee, for your continued support and involvement in this work. The worst Ebola outbreak in history *can* be stopped, and *will* be stopped. Thank you for enabling us to do everything we can to stop it. I look forward to your questions.

Mr. SMITH. Mr. Sedgewick, thank you very much for your testimony and your recommendations and, really, some of the good news, at least somewhat optimistic perspective, that you have provided the subcommittee.

Dr. Mans, please proceed.

STATEMENT OF DARIUS MANS, PH.D., PRESIDENT, AFRICARE

Mr. MANS. Thank you, Mr. Chairman.

Let me start by thanking you and members of the committee for your strong commitment to this issue. I also really want to applaud my colleagues here for the tireless work that they are doing on the ground. I am honored to be here with them.

If I may, I would like to start by describing what Africare is doing on the ground in the fight against Ebola and then describe to you what we at Africare believe are the most important steps that need to be taken in order to win this war.

It will be won by Africans on the ground who time and again have demonstrated that they can overcome disease and adversity. And, finally, I would like to conclude with what we believe the United States can do to stop Ebola in its tracks.

When the Ebola crisis began earlier this year, Africare immediately swung into action. We mobilized more than $2 million in private donations to help break the chain of transmission. We have shipped personal protection equipment and essential health supplies to all three affected countries through partnerships with Direct Relief and others. In addition, we have been helping frontline health workers do contact tracing.

Throughout the crisis, we have been very focused on community mobilization and behavior change. That is at the heart of what Africare does across the continent. We believe, while aid from foreign governments and from organizations like ours is vitally important, it will be Africans adopting changes in behavior that ultimately will win the war on the ground against Ebola.

So far, we have trained more than 300 local community health workers. They, in turn, have educated more than 150,000 Liberians about Ebola prevention, detection, and care.

In addition, our team of nearly 100 staff on the ground, all Liberian, are joined at the hip with Liberia's Ministry of Health to keep health facilities open to treat non-Ebola-related diseases, and that includes safe deliveries of babies. We are taking into our maternal waiting homes women who have been turned away from hospitals that are just overwhelmed by the Ebola crisis.

And since we believe that measurement is absolutely critical, we are also working with technology partners to find ways to embed data capture within our delivery systems so that we can provide good metrics to gauge our performance and real-time information about what we are doing to contribute to the war against Ebola. And I should tell you we are doing all of this without any funding from the U.S. Government so far.

But let me describe what we believe in addition needs to be done in the face of this challenge. Progress is being made, but much, much more needs to be done.

We certainly strongly support the President's emergency request and hope the rest of the G20 countries will step up to the plate and do more. But it is not just more money that is needed. It is important how that money is used.

There is a need for better coordination and planning of these emergency treatment centers. We believe we clearly don't need as many ETCs as were originally planned in Liberia, for example.

Very important to take the efforts to control Ebola to the community level. That is where the bulk of care is provided by family members, by neighbors, by local health workers who really are the first responders in this crisis.

We also hope that USAID will be given the flexibility to allocate its resources as needed to ensure there will be an agile response to what we have seen as a rapidly evolving epidemic.

And, in addition, very important, we believe that it is essential that civil society in the effected countries be given the support and space needed to help ensure the best use of an accountability for Ebola funding.

Finally, Mr. Chairman, let me say a few words about what more we believe the United States can do.

One of the big lessons of this crisis is that donors need to move beyond the old approach of vertical programming, of targeting resources to specific diseases like malaria and HIV/AIDS, as important that those are.

We need to invest in strengthening public health systems, especially community-based management of diseases. We also need to take advantage of this crisis to build the health infrastructure that the affected countries will need for the future. The investments being made now during the crisis need to help them build more robust and resilient health systems.

As the Liberian President has said, we must ensure that everything we do now is not just with the aim of ending the outbreak, but to ensure that we come out with a stronger, efficient healthcare system.

And, finally, Mr. Chairman, it is my hope that the U.S. Government will commit to support long-term economic growth in the region. I hope you will join me in urging the Millennium Challenge Corporation to quickly finalize its programs in Liberia and in Sierra Leone. Its significant investments in the key drivers for growth will be what is needed to help these countries get back on the higher growth path that they were on before the Ebola crisis.

Thank you, Mr. Chairman.

[The prepared statement of Mr. Mans follows:]

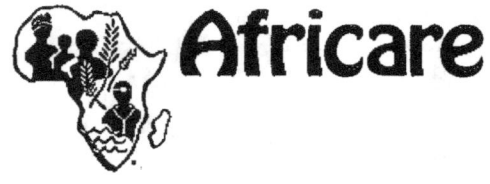

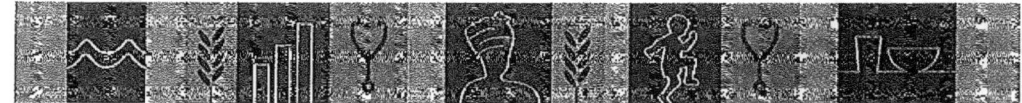

WITNESS

Darius Mans, Ph.D.
President
Africare

HOUSE COMMITTEE ON FOREIGN AFFAIRS
Subcommittee on Africa, Global Health, Global Human Rights, and International
Organizations

"Fighting Ebola: A Ground-Level View"

November 18, 2014

Darius Mans, President of AFRICARE

House Committee on Foreign Affairs

November 18, 2014

Fighting Ebola: A Ground-Level View

Thank you Mr. Chairman,

Let me start by thanking you and the Members of the Committee for your very strong commitment and leadership.

I also really want to applaud the heroic efforts of International Medical Corps and Global Communities who I am truly honored to be here with today.

Thank you for seeking the views from the "ground" and the opportunity to share Africare's perspective from having been on the ground now for 45 years, standing with thousands of communities across 36 countries in Africa.

Mr. Chairman, if I may, first I would like to very briefly describe what Africare has been doing in its fight against Ebola.

Then I'd like to lay out what we at Africare believe are the most important steps that need to be taken to win this war, which will be won by Africans on the ground who have, time and again, demonstrated that they can overcome disease and adversity.

And finally, I will conclude with what we believe the United States can do to stop Ebola in its tracks.

AFRICARE and EBOLA

When the Ebola crisis began earlier this year in West Africa, Africare immediately swung into action.

We mobilized more than $2 million in private donations to help break the chain of transmission.

We have shipped personal protection equipment and essential health supplies to Sierra Leone, Guinea and Liberia through partnerships with Direct Relief and local aid organizations.

In addition, we have been helping frontline health workers do contact tracing.

Throughout the crisis we have been very focused on community mobilization and behavior change, which is at the heart of what Africare does across the continent.

While aid from foreign governments and private voluntary contributions from organizations like ours is vitally important, it will be Africans adopting changes in behavior that will ultimately win the war on the ground against Ebola.

So far, we have trained more than 300 local volunteer community health workers.

They, in turn, have educated more than 150,000 Liberians about Ebola prevention, detection and care.

In addition, our team of nearly 100 staff on the ground—all Liberian—are joined at the hip with the Liberia Ministry of Health to help keep health facilities open to treat non-Ebola related diseases.

This includes ensuring safe deliveries of babies.

We are taking into our maternal waiting homes women who have been turned away from hospitals that are simply overwhelmed by the Ebola crisis.

We believe that measurement is critical.

We are talking with technology partners to find ways to embed data capture within our delivery systems.

We want to be sure we have good metrics to gauge our performance and provide real-time information on what we are doing to contribute to the war against Ebola.

And, we are doing all of this without any funding from the US Government so far.

WHAT MORE NEEDS TO BE DONE

Mr. Chairman, members of the Committee, progress is being made.

But much, much more needs to be done.

We strongly support the President's emergency request and hope the rest of the G20 countries will step up to the plate and do more.

But it's not just more **money** that is needed.

It's also important **how** that money is used.

There is a need for better coordination and planning of ETCs.

We also clearly don't need as many ETCs as originally planned in Liberia.

We believe it is vital that the efforts to control Ebola are taken to the community level.

That is where the bulk of the care is provided--by family members, neighbors and local health workers who really are the first responders in this crisis.

We also hope USAID will be given the flexibility to allocate its resources as needed to ensure an agile response to this rapidly evolving epidemic.

In addition, we believe it is essential that civil society in the affected countries be given the support and space needed to help ensure the best use of, and accountability for, Ebola funding .

Finally, let me say a few words about WHAT MORE CAN THE UNITED STATES DO ?

One of the big lessons of this crisis is that donors need to move beyond the old approach of targeting resources to specific disease burdens like malaria and HIV/AIDS.

We need to invest in strengthening the public health systems and especially community-based management of diseases.

We also need to take advantage of the crisis to build the health infrastructure the affected countries need in the future.

The investments being made now during the crisis need to help the affected countries build more robust and resilient health systems.

As Liberian President Johnson-Sirleaf said, "We must ensure that everything we do now is not just with the aim of ending the outbreak but to ensure that we come out with a stronger and efficient healthcare system."

Furthermore, it is my hope that the USG will commit to long-term economic growth in the region.

I hope you will join me in urging the Millennium Challenge Corporation to quickly finalize its programs in Liberia and Sierra Leone.

Significant investments in the key drivers for growth in those countries will help them get back onto the higher growth path they were on before the great disruption of the Ebola crisis.

Thank you Mr. Chairman for the opportunity to share Africare's views

Mr. SMITH. Thank you. Dr. Mans, thank you very much for the extremely valuable work you are doing, but, also, the insight you provide our committee.

Let me ask you a couple of questions, to all three of you.

You mentioned, Dr. Mans, that you have 300 local volunteer community health workers that you have trained who, in turn, have educated some 150,000 Liberians about Ebola prevention, detection, and care.

In your statement, Mr. Torbay, you talked about the need to ensure the availability of adequate, well-trained, well-protected healthcare workers.

How close are Liberia, Guinea, and Sierra Leone to having an optimum number of healthcare workers who are adequately trained? What is the deficit?

I mean, this is excellent information and very encouraging information. Are you finding people have been scared away because of the fear of contracting it themselves?

So if you could provide that information to us.

Secondly, Mr. Sedgewick—which I would point out parenthetically we are both from New Jersey. Welcome.

You talked about how the safe body management is of the highest priority to stopping the spread of Ebola, and you mentioned the CDC number of up to 70 percent of cases originating from contact from the deceased.

I think a lot of people are not unaware, but they have not known how stark the transmission is at that period of time when somebody has passed away. And you have very good information about your teams reaching 96 percent of bodies within 24 hours over the last month.

How many of the folks that should be reached are not being reached, just to try to get a sense of the unmet need? And what is the role that clergy and church are playing?

Obviously, when somebody passes away, we all turn to our faith. The church plays a key role, obviously, in funerals.

What role are they playing from the pulpit and in any other way of getting that message out about the contagious nature of someone who is deceased from Ebola?

With regard to personal protective equipment, Mr. Torbay, that is the third point that you made—how available is it, especially to those volunteers and those indigenous individuals who might not have access to it, as some of the NGOs do, going in? If you could just speak to that. Are we where we should be? Anywhere close to it? Because, obviously, that is one way of protecting.

And then, Dr. Mans, you had mentioned, and rightfully so, the deep concern of President Sirleaf. When I spoke to her, she raised the concern, and you have echoed her concern here today, about other diseases that continue to have a devastating impact on people in the three affected countries, including Liberia.

Congratulations and good work on the safe delivery aspect, to help both mother and baby have a venue where they can give birth as safely as possible. You might want to expand upon that.

How many women are we talking about who have gotten help through your work?

I have other questions, but I will ask those first and then yield to my friend and colleague and then come back for a few others.

Mr. TORBAY. Thank you, Mr. Chairman, for your questions.

I will start with the health workers gap. What we are doing at the International Medical Corps is focusing on training health workers that will be working in Ebola treatment units. That training is a 14-day intensive training that includes hands-on training actually treating patients in an Ebola treatment unit.

As you probably know, when you work in an Ebola treatment unit, you cannot work for more than an hour or, maximum, 2 before you get out because of the heat, because of the pressure, because of the stress, and we want to make sure that those workers go out before they get tired and dehydrated because this is when mistakes happen. So we are extremely careful about that.

In terms of the healthcare gap, we are coordinating with agencies that are doing community work, such as, you know, Global Communities, Africare, Samaritan's Purse, and other groups as well, and the idea is to combine and coordinate the community-based approach with the treatment-based approach because one cannot work properly or be effective without the other.

As you know, Liberia and Sierra Leone, even before Ebola, had very low doctor-per-patient ratios. We are talking 1 doctor for 100,000 in Liberia, and that is before 324 health workers have died from Ebola. So you can just imagine the gap.

One thing that is critical to the health gap, we cannot be only reactive. Anytime there is an outbreak, this is when we decide to train. We need to build a stronger healthcare system. We need to build a stronger preparedness system in all of these countries. And we need to focus on health workforce development.

Again, it is not just the infectious diseases. It is the malaria. It is the safe delivery. It is diarrhea. It is vaccine-preventable diseases that children are dying from.

I think we are on track in terms of training health workers for the Ebola response, but what we are doing in our Ebola training facilities is that we will be turning it in the next couple of months to an infectious disease academy that covers much more beyond Ebola.

And this is the sustainability aspect that we are encouraging all of our colleagues to look at, what comes beyond Ebola.

Mr. SMITH. Mr. Sedgewick.

Mr. SEDGEWICK. Thank you for your question.

To address your second question on unmet need, I would like to point out that the 96 percent of bodies that are collected within 24 hours, that is within 24 hours of the death of the individual, not of the phone call. So much of that 4 percent is because of a delay between the death and the phone call and the assignment of the team.

That is a big effort that we are working on in terms of our social mobilization and the social mobilization that all of the other partners are doing to ensure that that phone call happens very early on. Ideally, we are hearing about the status of the individual well before they pass.

As much as possible, our success is made significantly easier by our colleagues, like IMC, running ETUs and having the volume and the beds available to treat those individuals. It is much better for the individual to first get community care and then get to the ETU, that allows our teams to do a lot less work, which is a great situation to be in.

In terms of the larger question of unmet need, it is very difficult to understand. We do a lot of work with the communities, trying to understand if there are people dying that are getting hidden, and it is all anecdotal.

I know that the African Union and the CDC have been working on doing some studies on this and they found limited volumes of people hiding, but any are devastating.

So we are really working on making sure that the stigma goes down, which would encourage everyone to call and to reduce that unmet need.

In terms of volume, we are completely mobilized and we are able to respond very quickly. We have mobilized new teams within a day. So we are able to make sure that, as hot spots come up, the teams are positioned and available and responding immediately.

On the second part of that question regarding clergy and faith-based leaders, they are a core part of how we interact with the communities. Our historical interactions in Liberia have been focused on Bong, Lofa, and Nimba Counties. And so we have really strong relationships not just with the religious leaders, but with the traditional leaders and with the health leaders.

That made our initial entry with burial teams fairly straightforward. You can't drive one of our vehicles through those counties without getting stopped and having them ask how is so-and-so and how is so-and-so's baby. They are so engaged there that it made it very, very straightforward.

When we moved to other counties, especially in the southeast where we have less of a historical presence, we very quickly realized that we had to do really extensive interactions with religious, health, and traditional leaders, and they have been incredibly helpful in making sure that the communities know why we are there, that we are there for a good reason, that we are helping, and that we are able to do our work respectfully, closely, and rapidly. And so that has been a core part.

The religious leaders have been really helpful, and the traditional leaders, who also serve very important roles at the community level, have been very important for making sure that our teams are able to operate rapidly and safely.

Mr. SMITH. Thank you.

Mr. MANS. On personal protection equipment, no, we are nowhere near where we need to be. There are shortages of all kinds of equipment, including gloves for medical personnel to use.

So what Africare is doing is working with the private sector here in the United States, the big suppliers of equipment, like J&J and so many others, to be sure that we can get a steady supply of consumables into all health facilities in Liberia, working with all of the NGO partners, because we are a big believer in collaboration, that no one of us can do this alone.

And, second, on safe motherhood, you may know even before the Ebola crisis Liberia had one of the highest rates of maternal mortality in the world and headed in the wrong direction, increasing.

So a big focus for us has been in building more and more of these maternal waiting homes and working with the private sector in Liberia to raise the money to do so. So far, I think we are up to about 20.

And in these facilities, the point is to bring access to communities because women who were expecting were not able to get to these health facilities, which are so few and far between. And that is something we intend to continue to do post-crisis.

Mr. SMITH. Thank you.

Ms. BASS.

Ms. BASS. I again want to thank all of you for your testimony. I think it has been extremely helpful. And I have questions for each of you.

Mr. Torbay, in your recommendations, the second one says you wanted to make sure that the construction of the ETUs are appropriate for the needs of each country.

And so I was wondering if you find what is going on now is not appropriate. You know, are you saying this in response to something that needs to be improved?

Mr. TORBAY. Thank you for your question. That is actually a very important question, and we have been discussing it over the past week.

There had been plans to build a certain number of ETUs in every country based on findings that are about 2 months old.

The situation is evolving rapidly, and we need to make sure that, as it evolves, we do not stick to the old plans, that actually we adapt and we are flexible enough so that if there is no need for an ETU, let's not even build that ETU.

If there is a need for mobile teams that would go out and get patients to an Ebola treatment unit that has empty beds, let's do that, because we are seeing some Ebola treatment units that have an overflow of patients and some Ebola treatments units——

Ms. BASS. They are empty.

Mr. TORBAY [continuing]. That actually have empty beds.

Ms. BASS. Right.

Mr. TORBAY. And we need to make sure that we balance that.

Ms. BASS. I heard about that, too, and I had thought that one of the reasons was because the population was, you know, afraid to come forward and the best case is that they are not needed, but that that wasn't the issue.

So why do you have that discrepancy? And then I guess what you are saying is why Dr. Mans was saying that maybe ETUs is not the way to go right now.

But I will come back to you, Dr. Mans.

Mr. TORBAY. Well, first of all, the virus is moving. It is not staying in one county. So you build an Ebola treatment unit in one county. You get it under control with the work between the community-based approach and the treatment approach.

It is getting under control, but then it is appearing in another country——

Ms. BASS. Right.

Mr. TORBAY [continuing]. In another county. So that is why there are large numbers in certain areas and lower numbers. And those need to be coordinated.

And we support the community approach because, at the end of the day, Ebola started at the community level and this where it should die, at the community level.

Ms. Bass. Right.

Mr. Torbay. And we need to make sure that the community centers are well equipped and the staff are well trained to detect and isolate so they could refer to the treatment units for further treatments and those that are negative could be discharged back into the community. And this is what needs strengthening, and this is the work that is being done now on the ground.

Ms. Bass. So you know how I said in my opening that I was interested to know if any of the things that we were building: Should they stay? I have not been inside an ETU. I have just seen them on TV.

Is there any value to the ETUs that were being built being left there for either other infectious diseases or other health needs?

Mr. Torbay. You know, some of those ETUs are not built to last——

Ms. Bass. Okay.

Mr. Torbay [continuing]. Which is fair enough. They are built with temporary material that would last for a few months, and that is good enough.

But one of the approaches we are following is we are trying to build a more permanent structure that could be later on turned into something else. It could be turned into a training center or a clinic. And that is the sustainable aspect of it, and that is what we are encouraging.

There will be a need for isolation wards or isolation units in west Africa that need to remain there even after we contain Ebola because chances are there might be other diseases, or Ebola might resurface, and there is a need for the facility as well as equipment and trained staff there.

Ms. Bass. So it was the first time I have heard someone talk about that the only time a healthcare worker can be with a patient is 1 to 2 hours.

Now, I have seen the equipment and I have seen the stories that talk about the heat, but that implies a large number of healthcare workers.

So if you are only with the patient, you know, for an hour or 2 and you leave, then do you have relief? Do you understand what I am saying?

Mr. Torbay. Absolutely.

Ms. Bass. So how does it work?

Mr. Torbay. In our Ebola treatment unit in Bong County in Liberia, it is a 70-bed treatment facility. We have 230 staff members working there.

Ms. Bass. Wow. Okay.

Mr. Torbay. We work around the clock. So it is by shifts.

Ms. Bass. I got it.

Mr. Torbay. When a doctor goes out, another one will be in to replace him.

Ms. Bass. And so, when the person leaves after being there an hour or 2, they take a break of how long? And then I imagine they go back for——

Mr. TORBAY. Yes. It really depends on the level of exhaustion and dehydration. Usually, it is not less than 3 to 4 hours. They need to recover before we bring them back in.

Ms. BASS. Wow. Okay.

And, Dr. Mans, maybe you could respond to this one if you wanted to add anything about the ETUs. But, also, I know that there was an issue around the healthcare workers at one point and them being paid and them wanting hazard pay, and I was wondering what the situation was with that, if that has improved.

Mr. MANS. Sure. Thank you, ma'am.

You know, I agree completely with what Rabih has just said about the ETCs as part of the strategy.

Ms. BASS. ETCs.

Mr. MANS. Emergency treatment centers. Sorry.

And there are some certainly challenges around planning and coordination. For example, we have seen, you know, the United States Government construct a 100-bed emergency treatment center, you know, 3 miles from where MSF is operating one. The Chinese Government has built one in between. And, yet, communities where there are hot spots not very far away, but not accessible easily by road, can't get into any of those. So, again——

Ms. BASS. So how does that happen?

Mr. MANS [continuing]. The challenge of planning, coordination——

Ms. BASS. How does that happen?

Mr. MANS [continuing]. Is what is very important.

Fundamentally, it is a responsibility of government.

And so I think finding ways, again, as Rabih, I think, summed up so well, making sure that there is a more mobile response to be able to get people into the facilities where they need support.

Because what worries me in this is the gap that I see in talking to Liberians about these big numbers that they hear that has been committed to Ebola and the actual response that is taking place on the ground.

And so I think it is extremely important to be sure that the planning is done effectively, that that communication is out there, so that citizens', in these countries, expectations can be better managed.

The other thing I just wanted to add is about training, which was discussed earlier, which I think is extremely important. We think a lot about it; we work with community health workers and, of course, there is a big challenge.

There are so few doctors in Liberia. Just take one example: 4 million people, 425 doctors. But it is a big challenge, I think, to provide not just more training for medical personnel, but some of this pre-service training at the technical level is desperately needed and could be done pretty quickly.

And I think that there are institutions here in the United States that can provide the kind of support that is needed to ramp up pre-service training as well as supporting in-service training by institutions in the affected countries.

Ms. BASS. Now, both of you or maybe all of you made reference to we need to take it to the community and have the community be involved. And I wanted to know if maybe you could be specific about that.

I certainly understand the community piece in terms of the contact tracing, identifying, people that are infected.

And then what? If there are not ETCs, ETUs, whatever, then what? So you are taking it to the community, you have identified a person. Then what? You follow me?

Mr. TORBAY. I can try to answer that.

The role of the community is critical. As you mentioned, contact tracing is critical. Informing the authorities is also very important, informing burial teams so they could remove the body.

But also very important is to educate the community about what to do if they see someone presenting with symptoms, how to isolate that person and make sure that also they have at least gloves or things to protect themselves, but to make sure that they isolate and inform the different authorities, be it the health workers or the community health workers.

This is critical because what is happening is that there are people that have Ebola that are staying in the same room with five other people, and that cannot happen. The isolation is critical and this is where the education at the community level becomes very important because that is the only way we can contain it.

Ms. BASS. So should there be smaller ETCs? Because I understand isolating the person. But if you isolate the person without treatment, the person is just going to sit there and die.

Then you said that the ETCs are maybe in inappropriate places or maybe they are not needed. But in the places where they are not needed, then what happens to the person?

Mr. TORBAY. That is a very valid question.

There are community care centers that are being established, which are like mini Ebola treatment centers.

Ms. BASS. Okay.

Mr. TORBAY. And the idea is those patients will be taken there. They will be isolated. They will be cared for until the test is done. Then they are referred. So the important thing is for them to be taken out of their home.

And I would just like to add one thing as well that you mentioned initially about the U.S. Government and the ETCs.

In our discussion with the U.S. military, as well as with USAID, about the need for Ebola treatment units and where they should be, we have seen that they have been extremely flexible and receptive.

So if we tell them, "Hey, there is no need for us to staff this one. Let's move it there," they have been extremely responsive to recommendations. And I would like to commend them for that.

Ms. BASS. Okay. And, Mr. Sedgewick, you might want to respond, but I wanted to ask you a series of questions around cultural practices. But go ahead and respond.

Mr. SEDGEWICK. Yeah. I would like to catch up a little bit and I would like to reiterate that flexibility on both the designation of where the ETUs are and, in general, that flexibility that, in particular, the USAID DART, and the general response has been really fantastic and it has allowed us to make sure that we are able to position resources as quickly as possible.

On the issue of the community, we spend a lot of time and have spent a lot of time since April going over what the best way is to interact with the community, and that is a lot of these dialogue sessions that I have been talking about.

It is really focused on making sure that we are not top-down, we are not distributing leaflets and just doing radio shows, though we are doing that, but really making sure that it is a conversation with the community about what Ebola is and what it is not and having them come up with their own solutions that we work through.

And that has been able to allow us to make sure that the communities, when they have a suspected case, that they put the community member in a separate location, that the communities are doing a lot of their own monitoring, and making sure that they are making that phone call.

Really, that phone call is the most important thing, making sure that that victim or suspected victim is isolated. Them making that phone call is really huge.

In the long term, before we started, before this fire hit, we were doing these water and sanitation activities with the government and we were successful in working with over 350 communities in Bong, Lofa, and Nimba on proper sanitation and proper hygiene. And that effort was incredibly successful.

In all 350 communities, in Bong, Lofa, and Nimba, which are some of the hardest hit communities, none of them have been affected by Ebola.

And it really goes to show that, if you make that long-term investment, if you prepare the communities before it hits, it has a huge impact and it really prevents that from happening. And I only wish that we were able to hit all the communities in Liberia before the virus hit.

Ms. BASS. So I wanted to ask if you would expand a little bit more.

You were talking about the cultural practices. And I do understand—first of all, it was really something when you said that 70 percent of the transmissions were due to contact with people who had passed away.

How long is a body contagious?

And then my colleague was asking about the role of the faith community. And I was just wondering if faith leaders—since, obviously, the traditions are a part of people's faith, if they were taking the lead in getting people to deviate, to divert, from traditional practices. And I would imagine that would be really hard.

You said that they have come up with ways to safely say good-bye, and I thought you said that they did that with all of the protective gear on. And I was wondering if that is what you meant.

And then, finally, I want to know what happened to you. You were there. You came back. Did they hold you in a tent at the airport? I mean, I am glad they didn't, if they didn't. But how did you sneak back in?

Mr. SEDGEWICK. Great. Well, thank you. And that is a series of great questions.

I will answer the last one first. I was met at the airport. There was an "X" on my piece of paper as I was trying to get out——

Ms. BASS. Seriously?

Mr. SEDGEWICK [continuing]. You know, that pulled me over to the side. And so I conducted an interview with the CDC.

Ms. BASS. What airport?

Mr. SEDGEWICK. Dulles.

And they were really great. They streamlined the process as quickly as possible, asked me about my potential level of exposure, which was very limited, and took my temperature.

And, since then, I have been in daily contact with the DC Department of Health. I live in DC, so that I am in contact them every day. I self-monitor, take my temperature twice a day, and monitor any symptoms, of which I have none.

But I would like to reiterate that they, the CDC and the DC Department of Health, are really focused on the partnership aspect of it and the fact that we are working together on this and that they understand why I am there and why I went and that it is not an antagonistic relationship, that we work together.

And that allows not just me, but everyone coming back, to feel free and happy to discuss our health with the Department of Health and with the CDC, and that really opens up that dialogue. It makes it, I think, much more impactful in terms of a monitoring tool.

On your question about safely saying goodbye, we don't allow the community members to don PPEs as a prevention tool because it requires a lot of training. We do actually, though, allow them to don some PPEs to make them feel better because, honestly, the burial teams are wearing full PPEs. It is fairly intimidating.

And so, if it makes them feel better to wear some PPEs, we allow them to do that, but we don't allow them anywhere near the body. And they have to——

Ms. BASS. So it was the burial teams you were describing?

Mr. SEDGEWICK. Yeah. The burial teams are wearing the full PPEs. The community members are allowed to attend the burial and, if they want to, they can wear some limited PPEs, but, really, they are not allowed close.

But that allows them to understand what is happening, where the burial is, to watch the process, which is incredibly important, to make sure that they are engaged and to make sure that the next time there is a victim, that they make that phone call.

So that interaction really takes the bulk of the time. The way that the burial teams interact with the communities and make sure the burial is done in a respectful and dignified way is a huge part of their time.

The other small item that I wanted to respond to was on the hazard pay, which is a really important aspect of the response, actually. Because these are really brave people doing really important work, but they do want to make sure that they are being compensated.

And so that is a part of our efforts, is to make sure that that pay is happening on time and really working to ensure that. It is a small amount of money by our standards, but it is incredibly important to make sure that they understand that they are valued and that the work that they are doing is important.

Ms. BASS. Just quickly to the two last questions, which were how long is a body contagious——

Mr. SEDGEWICK. Oh. I'm sorry. Yes.

Ms. BASS [continuing]. And then if somebody could address the abandoned children. Where are they? What is happening to them?

Mr. SEDGEWICK. Sure.

On the length of time that a body is contagious, we don't exactly know. And the CDC and the WHO are looking at this. And so that is why we are just focused on—it is a long time.

It is on the order of weeks. And so that is why we make sure that the body is, you know, covered in chlorine, placed in a body bag, covered in chlorine again when it is buried.

It is alternating soil and chlorine so that there is no risk. The virus doesn't last very long in water even. So it is very low risk to the water tables. But we also make sure that burials happen above the water table just to make sure.

Ms. BASS. Thank you.

Mr. SMITH. Thank you.

Just a few follow-up questions.

At our September 17 hearing, Dr. Kent Brantly from Samaritan's Purse spoke at length about a number of things, having lived through it and having survived. One point that he made was that the 120-bed isolation unit at his hospital, ELWA, was turning away as many as 30 infectious individuals each day.

And I am wondering, with the ETUs, has that changed or is the capacity growing? The military certainly is in the process, and you might give an update on how well you think the United States military is doing in creating that capacity.

He also made a very strong point about those who will stay in their home and will be cared for by loved ones, husbands, wives, children. He said, "If we do not provide education and protective equipment to caregivers, we will be condemning countless numbers of mothers, fathers, daughters, and sons to death simply because they chose not to let their loved ones die alone."

And I'm wondering, since, obviously, isolation is one of the keys to breaking the transmission chain and many of these infected people will stay at home, is the outreach to the individual caregivers as robust as it should be?

Let me also ask, at the second hearing, Dr. Fauci from NIH used the word "exponential" time and time again during his testimony. We had a group of top people, including the head of USAID, at a hearing last week of the full committee, and that word wasn't uttered once. And I asked them, "Are we seeing a turn?"

You know, CDC had said that, if the rate of increase continues at the pace in September, there could be as many as 1.4 million cases by late January. Where are we, in your view, in terms of the estimations of how large this epidemic may grow?

Let me also ask you about one of the 10 points that you have suggested to us, Mr. Torbay, the importance of a capable ambulance network.

And I am wondering, since so many people can't get to an ETU or any other kind of health facility, where is Liberia, and perhaps the other two countries as well, but I think you know more about Liberia, in terms of ambulance capacity?

And, also, if I could, all of you might want to touch on this. You know, Dr. Brantly may have been helped by ZMapp. We still don't know. There are other drugs still in the pipeline, vaccines and curative potential drugs.

I was amazed and positively shocked when you said, Mr. Torbay, that the rate of fatality at your Bong County Ebola unit in Liberia is approximately 26 percent. That is far lower than the average fatality rate in the three affected countries.

And I am wondering, what is being done there to achieve those remarkable results in terms of mitigating fatality? So if you could speak to those issues.

Mr. TORBAY. Thank you, Mr. Chairman.

I would like to start with the last question about the low fatality rate at our Ebola treatment unit in Bong.

We are not using any miraculous drug or any testing drug there. What we are doing is working with the community to make sure that patients are referred to the Ebola treatment unit as soon as possible. That has been one of the major factors in lowering mortality rates.

And as you have seen even here in the U.S., those that were caught early on and sent to the hospital, they survived, and those that were late did not make it, unfortunately. And, for us, that is extremely important.

Our treatment is very basic. It is palliative care. It is hydration. It is balance of electrolytes. It is making sure that people actually are healthy enough for them to fight the virus on their own.

One very critical component of, actually, our success has been the U.S. Navy lab that was set up right next to our Ebola treatment unit. It used to take us 5 to 7 days before we would get the test results for a suspect case. Now it takes us 5 to 7 hours.

So, basically, people are coming in. We are testing them. If they are positive, they are put in the treatment ward. If they are negative, they are sent home. And that cuts down on the potential exposure as well. This has been critical for us as well.

Mr. SMITH. Excuse me.

That would be of people manifesting some symptom?

Mr. TORBAY. Correct.

Mr. SMITH. Okay.

Mr. TORBAY. Correct. They manifest symptoms. They are put as a suspect case until they are tested. Then we decide whether it is positive or negative.

Mr. SMITH. And if they are not manifesting a symptom, no testing is done?

Mr. TORBAY. No.

Mr. SMITH. Okay.

Mr. TORBAY. This actually ties into your question about the Ebola treatment unit capacity. Actually, the lab facilities are playing a critical role because the Ebola treatment units accept suspect cases. And that is why they were turning a lot of cases away, because they did not have the capacity to test a lot of those patients. They have to keep them there until they are tested.

So with the additional number of labs that are being established in Liberia and Sierra Leone, that is helping out and it is no longer the case. Hardly any unit is actually pushing patients away. The situation in Liberia, and this is something that Dr. Shah, I think, mentioned here in his testimony, is looking better than it looked a couple of months ago. The numbers are lower. The new cases are lower than it was before. It is much better than what we estimated 2 months ago. And if we continue on the right track—and we have to continue with the same momentum, we cannot slow down—we will get it under control.

And the same applies for the other countries. Liberia—now we see the numbers in Sierra Leone, actually, are increasing at a much faster rate than Liberia. So we need to work together—community, the treatment, the host government, as well as donors and other governments and the military—to contain it. And Liberia could be a really good success story.

Now, we shouldn't start celebrating yet. We have to be very careful. It is still not under control. It is looking positive. If we continue, we will get it under control, but it is too early to actually start celebrating.

On the individual family protection, this is something that is definitely important. This goes back to educating the family, but also giving them basic protection equipment, gloves, mask.

But at the same time, we do not want to give them a false sense of protection. We do not want them to think that, just because they have gloves and a mask, they are okay to be near a patient. We need to make sure that the education takes place properly and that they are very well aware of the risks even with the protection. And that is very critical.

Ambulance network. That is very important in all three countries. And, you know, we turned pickup trucks into ambulances. We turned anything that we could get our hands on into ambulances. We are looking at different types of ambulances, including air ambulances that could take patients from faraway counties into our Ebola treatment units. It is much better and much cheaper than setting up another Ebola treatment unit in some of those counties.

There is a need to increase that capacity, and there is also a need to train staff working in ambulances because that is a very risky job when you are in an ambulance. It seems that there is a move now to actually get ambulances in there. There are a lot of ambulances being donated. We are buying a lot of ambulances. Also, we look at alternative ways of transportation.

Mr. MANS. Yes. If I may, I just wanted to add to Rabih's point about getting to that inflection point on the Ebola crisis.

I think this combination of getting both the hardware right and the software right, hugely important. One, these ETCs and getting many ETCs out into communities, getting community care centers to improve access.

On the other side is what I see happening on the technology front and very quickly so that we are in a position to do a better job of testing, tracking, and treating the virus.

On the testing side, a number of rapid diagnostic tests are becoming available, being tested out on the ground in the next couple of months.

A lot of work is being done with U.S.-based technology companies working with people on the ground to develop tools to automate contact tracing, to bring the power of technology into this to be able to do a much better job of tracking and doing surveillance.

I think that, too, is coming in addition to what is happening on the treatment side. So like my colleagues, I am very hopeful, but we cannot be complacent or declare victory. There is still a lot of work to be done on all these fronts.

Mr. SEDGEWICK. I would like to go through a few of your questions because I think they are really interesting and show the changes, especially in reference to Dr. Brantly's testimony.

I believe there was sort of a vicious cycle that was going on at the early stages where there was not enough testing. So there were not enough beds. And so Ebola patients were being turned away from the ETUs both because of the lack of testing and just the simple lack of beds and healthcare workers.

And so then the victims are turned away. They go back into their community and they infect others and they pass away. And the burial teams at that point were overstretched.

And so both of those issues being addressed—the ETUs having the available beds and then the burial teams being able to collect all the bodies—really had a significant impact on lowering the rate of transmission.

And then that cycle continued to bring down the number of Ebola victims going into the ETUs. So that has been one of the big flips that has happened since Dr. Brantly testified, which is, you know, wonderful to hear, obviously.

And I would like to reiterate that, while the communities do need protective equipment and do need education about how to handle the sick, that risk of the false sense of prevention that Mr. Torbay brought up is something that we are very careful about, that just because they have got a mask and gloves doesn't mean that they are going to be able to safely handle victims.

And, you know, the ETUs are not at all wasteful in terms of how they are put together. They are very straightforwardly put together. As he mentioned, most are temporary structures. And they are the fastest, lightest, high-quality treatment that you can get.

And so, as you move down from that, you do incur some risk, in terms of the community care centers, that have to be looked at very carefully to make sure that the quality of care at those ETCs are very, very high.

In terms of the projections that you mentioned, I think a lot of those projections were if nothing happened, if we don't do anything. So now that we are doing something—and I think we are doing a lot—that is bringing down a lot of those projections. And I think we will look forward to future projections as they come forward.

On the ambulance network, it is something that we are involved in in responding to. And we got into a lot of the other activities that we are doing, such as contact tracing and ambulance work and the community engagement work in the southeast, because we are locating our teams at the county health team. So we have a significant relationship with every county health team.

And we make sure that the burial teams are run out of that county health team. And so, when they say, "Hey, our ambulance broke down. Can you help us out?," we are able to immediately respond and very, very quickly to make sure that they have another ambulance or that their ambulance gets repaired. That has allowed us to engage about 10 ambulances that are being run out of different county health teams as they have requested it from us.

And I think that aspect of it—to make sure that we are hearing directly from the county health teams in some of these incredibly remote counties—some of them take 2 days to get to on a good, dry day—and we are able to hear from them immediately when they have these needs—allows us to respond very quickly.

I know Ranking Member Bass stepped out. But I think, on the orphan issue, it is a pretty significant issue that is being looked at by a lot of different NGOs. The entire question of how you respond to the families that are affected—orphans, widows, widowers—is really significant, and it is one of the lasting effects of this virus.

Mr. SMITH. Just let me conclude with these following questions.

Who is really in charge, like in Liberia? Is it the Ministry of Health? We know that WHO came under some withering criticism in mid-October from a report about how they had missed it and had inadequate staffing. I am just wondering, who is truly in charge? UNMEER, what role do they play? We know CDC is playing a very significant advisory and leadership role.

And, secondly, on the issue of training community healthcare workers, could you just give a sense what their ages are. Are they older, more experienced people who have come back into the system? Are they young people who are stepping up to the plate? I mean, what does that look like? And does USAID provide any kind of salary support?

We know that, in catastrophic situations, very often that kind of subsidy can be provided. I remember being in Sri Lanka after the tsunami, and we were paying salaries to individuals to do work, to do cleanup. And it not only was motivating, but they were actively doing the cleanup of their own homes and communities, and there was that significant subsidy to help them get money in their pocket to get their businesses going locally. And I am wondering if USAID or any other entity in government is providing any salary support.

Mr. TORBAY. The Liberian Government is in charge, and they should be in charge. At the end of the day, that is their country and we are just guests there. And we only work through them and with them. And I don't think any of those countries were prepared for such an outbreak and especially countries like Liberia and Sierra Leone that have suffered from a long civil war and they were trying to recover from that and they still haven't fully recovered, in addition to the other systemic issues within the health systems there.

The World Health Organization, CDC, and NGOs work to support the Liberian Minister of Health and Social Welfare, and they have people seconded to them. They have a body that coordinates the Ebola response, and they have people from different agencies supporting them.

One thing that we definitely—going back to your initial question about what needs to be done to make sure that we do not go back there, we cannot afford to go back to where we were before the Ebola outbreak in terms of systems in those governments. We need to build the systems much better than they were before because, as we saw, they weren't that effective.

One way to do it is actually to support the Liberian, Sierra Leonean, or the Guinean Government, the Ministries of Health, build their systems, train their staff, give them all the support that they need to move things forward. You know, they are doing what they can, given the limited capacity and capabilities that they have.

UNMEER is now playing a more robust role than they did a while ago. As I mentioned in my testimony, there still needs to be clarification in terms of who is responsible for what and who is coordinating what. That is very important. And I think, as discussions take place on the ground, that should be clarified.

I will answer briefly about the health workers. And I am sure my colleagues here would give you a more detailed answer.

Most of our health workers that are working with us, the majority of them are younger. They are college kids or people who went to school or are working in the market, but they are younger. And those are the ones that have been working with us mostly.

In terms of USAID support, USAID has been very generous with us and other NGOs working on the ground. Whatever we ask them for, including salaries for staff working at the community or at the Ebola treatment units, there hasn't been any hesitation.

I do not know what is going on in terms of support for the Liberian Government, who should be paying—or who is paying the incentives. But as far as we are concerned, they have been extremely generous and effective and very pragmatic in their approach.

Mr. SEDGEWICK. I would like to reiterate that the Government of Liberia, in general, is leading the effort and the Ministry of Health and Social Welfare in particular.

Tolbert Nyenswah, who is the Assistant Minister of Health and has been leading the incident management system, has been a really great coordinator of the effort in those meetings, which happen, I think, about three times a week, makes sure that everyone is on the same page.

That has been our approach, is to make sure that we are leveraging the resources that they have and supplementing what they have to make sure that we are successful and that they are successful. And doing so has allowed us to move very, very quickly and be very responsive, as I mentioned before.

That said, the other actors, especially the USAID DART, have been incredibly responsive and excellent at coordinating their efforts and their various arms. The DART has been a really incredible partner for us to make sure that, as the situation changes on the ground, we are able to move very, very quickly.

On the community health workers, the system in Liberia that existed before was for all the community health workers to actually be community health volunteers. So they were unpaid volunteers that received supplemental support in some way or other occasionally. And I believe that, depending on what the activity is, they are getting some limited level of support.

Certainly from our side, when we do activities, they do get some incentive payments. If they are able to bring—if they are able to achieve certain deliverables, then we do give them some payments occasionally. I don't know if they are receiving large-scale salary from the Ministry of Health at this point during the emergency.

Mr. MANS. The only thing I would add, again, as I said earlier, is the great frustration that exists within Liberia, this crisis and the gap between what people perceive is actually happening on the ground and these very big numbers that the public hears about.

The Government, the President in particular, has been very forceful in demanding that the Government be very focused on this agenda. As you may know, she just had a shakeup in the cabinet. She replaced the Minister of Health to be sure that she has the leadership in that ministry to see this thing through.

So there is no sense of complacency. Quite the opposite. They are leading and working very hard to ensure that there is a joined-up government approach on their side, just as the United States Government has taken a joined-up whole-of-government approach.

Mr. SMITH. Thank you.

Just to conclude, I mentioned in the outset that we had just introduced H.R. 5710, the Ebola Emergency Response Act, and many of you have provided insights as to what ought to be in there.

I would ask you to take a look at it to see if it covers all the bases, if you will, and if you could see your way clear, after you look at it, you know, to perhaps support it, because I do think we are talking about a sustainable problem that needs a sustainable response.

And, you know, the good work that our House Appropriations and Senate Appropriations Committees have done, particularly when the DOD asked for a reprogramming request that was huge, it was done without the slightest bit of hesitation.

But we need to have the authorizers, I think, as well making sure that we leave no stone unturned as well in mitigating and, hopefully, ending this crisis. So please take a look at the legislation, if you would.

Anything you would like to say before we conclude?

Mr. TORBAY. I would just like to thank you for your leadership and the leadership of the U.S. Government. We are very proud of what has been achieved so far and the continuous focus on resolving this issue. And, again, thank you for having us here today.

Mr. SMITH. Thank you.

Mr. SEDGEWICK. I would like to reiterate that thanks.

And the efforts that you see on the ground in Liberia in particular are really incredible, and a large volume of that is due to the leadership of the U.S. Government and the leadership of the subcommittee to make sure that it happens.

So it is truly inspiring when you are in Liberia seeing the response happen and seeing the effort, the impact that we are all having. So thank you.

Mr. MANS. And I want to thank you for your continued leadership long after these headlines fade, and they will, to be sure that everybody is focused on how to rebuild in Liberia the health sector and get these countries back on track. So thank you for your leadership, sir.

Mr. SMITH. Thank you so very much.

And, again, I want to thank you for your expertise, your tremendous leadership, the three of you. It is just remarkable.

And, that said, the hearing is adjourned.

[Whereupon, at 11:32 a.m., the subcommittee was adjourned.]

APPENDIX

MATERIAL SUBMITTED FOR THE RECORD

SUBCOMMITTEE HEARING NOTICE
COMMITTEE ON FOREIGN AFFAIRS
U.S. HOUSE OF REPRESENTATIVES
WASHINGTON, DC 20515-6128

Subcommittee on Africa, Global Health, Global Human Rights, and International Organizations

Christopher H. Smith (R-NJ), Chairman

November 18, 2014

TO: MEMBERS OF THE COMMITTEE ON FOREIGN AFFAIRS

You are respectfully requested to attend an OPEN hearing of the Committee on Foreign Affairs, to be held by the Subcommittee on Africa, Global Health, Global Human Rights, and International Organizations in Room 2172 of the Rayburn House Office Building (and available live on the Committee website at www.foreignaffairs.house.gov):

DATE: Tuesday, November 18, 2014

TIME: 10:00 a.m.

SUBJECT: Fighting Ebola: A Ground-Level View

WITNESSES: Mr. Rabih Torbay
Senior Vice President for International Operations
International Medical Corps

Mr. Brett Sedgewick
Technical Advisor for Food Security and Livelihoods
Global Communities

Darius Mans, Ph.D.
President
Africare

By Direction of the Chairman

The Committee on Foreign Affairs seeks to make its facilities accessible to persons with disabilities. If you are in need of special accommodations, please call 202/225-5021 at least four business days in advance of the event, whenever practicable. Questions with regard to special accommodations in general (including availability of Committee materials in alternative formats and assistive listening devices) may be directed to the Committee.

COMMITTEE ON FOREIGN AFFAIRS

MINUTES OF SUBCOMMITTEE ON _Africa, Global Health, Global Human Rights, and International Organizations_ HEARING

Day___ _Tuesday___ Date___ _November 18, 2014___ Room_ _2172 Rayburn HOB_

Starting Time __ _10:07 a.m.___ Ending Time __ _11:32 a.m.___

Recesses | _0_ | (___to ___)(___to ___)(___to ___)(___to ___)(___to ___)(___to ___)

Presiding Member(s)

Rep. Chris Smith

Check all of the following that apply:

Open Session ☑   Electronically Recorded (taped) ☑
Executive (closed) Session ☐   Stenographic Record ☑
Televised ☑

TITLE OF HEARING:

Fighting Ebola: A Ground-Level View

SUBCOMMITTEE MEMBERS PRESENT:

Rep. Mark Meadows, Rep. Randy Weber, Rep. Karen Bass

NON-SUBCOMMITTEE MEMBERS PRESENT: _(Mark with an * if they are not members of full committee.)_

HEARING WITNESSES: Same as meeting notice attached? Yes ☑ No ☐
(If "no", please list below and include title, agency, department, or organization.)

STATEMENTS FOR THE RECORD: _(List any statements submitted for the record.)_

TIME SCHEDULED TO RECONVENE _____
or
TIME ADJOURNED __ _11:32 a.m._

Gregory B. Simpkins
Subcommittee Staff Director

www.ingramcontent.com/pod-product-compliance
Lightning Source LLC
Chambersburg PA
CBHW081120280526
45787CB00007B/2916